CONTENTS

Introduction
What Are Essential Oils?   1
Young Living   9
Plant Therapy   11
Revive Essential Oils   13
Edens Garden   15
doTERRA   17
But before you begin…   19
Types of Essential Oils   20
Choosing the Right Essential Oils   38
Afterword   41

INTRODUCTION

Essential oil diffusers are the new "it" girl. Their calming therapeutic effects have hypnotized everyone and almost every home, office, school, shop, and even gym seems to have one. But what are essential oil diffusers and why are they so popular these days? We are here with a simple beginner's guide to essential oils to help you understand just how magical they are and whether or not they are worth the buck.

WHAT ARE ESSENTIAL OILS?

Essential oils are a sector of complementary and alternative medicine, or CAM, that are treatments outside of the immediate medical field. And as the market for CAM has increased in the past few years, so has people's interest in essential oils, diffusers, aromatherapy, and such. The Global Aromatherapy Market Analysis, Companies Profiles, Size, Share, Growth, Trends and Forecast predicts that the market for aromatherapy will grow by 8 percent by 2024.

Inhaling the aromas from essential oils can stimulate areas of your limbic system, which is a part of your brain that plays a role in emotions, behaviors, sense of smell, and long-term memory.

Healthline.com

So, what are these essential oils everyone is raving about? For our beginners who are new to this trend, essential oils are highly potent oils that come from plants. They have many beneficial properties and are available in various flavors/scents. They are multipurpose, so they can be used on your hair, on your skin, for aromatherapy, and few medical purposes too.

Where did essential oils come from? Though it might seem like essential oils are only now gaining popularity, the essential oil story began in ancient times, nearly 5,000 years ago, in Egypt, Persia, and India. As a matter of fact, many historians point to essential oils as one of the world's oldest forms of medication. The first recorded use of essential oils is dated around 4,500 B.C.E. Believing that the oils were sacred and pure, the Ancient Egyptians reserved the use of essential oils for priests. In fact, essential oils were closely integrated into their religious practices. The Egyptians assigned different essential oils to their various gods and believed that the oils could help win wars and calm the mind.

Ancient Egypt was well known for being technologically and medicinally advanced, mostly due to its prime location near the Nile River. The fertile soil that came with their geographical location allowed them to thrive economically, have an abundant (and permanent) supply of food, and transport people and goods whenever they saw fit. In short, the Nile River pushed the development of things like culture and medicine forward at an extremely fast rate, which meant that Ancient Egypt was the perfect birthplace for essential oils.

It wasn't long before the Ancient Egyptians utilized essential oils for medicinal purposes. Most notably, essential oils were used during the process of mummification, wherein the bodies of high-profile people like pharaohs were dried and preserved in preparation for the afterlife. Traces of aromatic cedar, juniper essential oil, and myrrh have recently been discovered in mummified bodies, which points to the fact that essential oils were used to keep the embalmed bodies cleansed, preserved, and desiccated. These oils were also buried with the bodies for spiritual purposes. Their potent aromas were meant to appease the apparitions in the afterlife and signify the status of the soul in question.

The world's first recorded chemist, a woman that went by the name of Tapputi, used essential oils such as myrrh and balsam in her practices. As recorded in a cuneiform tablet that originated from the ancient civilization of Mesopotamia and was dated back to around 1200 BC, Tapputi often incorporated the oils into the perfumes that she made. She is also known for being one of the first operators of a still, which is basically a huge distillation machine.

Another early use of essential oils occurred in the practice known as Ayurveda. Ayurveda, a Sanskrit word that translates to "The Science of Life," is an ancient Indian science mainly used in the realm of medicine and healing. Ayurveda focuses on balancing the energies of the body and is meant to serve as a complement to traditional Western medicine. Vedic culture has produced lists of various essential oils, such as ginger and cinnamon, that are meant to guide patients when it comes to healing their afflictions.

Essential oils were also an integral part of medicinal practices during Biblical times. Essential oils are mentioned in the Bible 188 times, and there are references to over 33 different oils and oil-producing plants. Though the most famous Biblical oils are frankincense and myrrh, both of which were brought, along with gold, to baby Jesus as gifts, the scripture lists many other highly revered oils. Spikenard, comparable to modern lavender oil, may have been used to anoint Jesus days before his crucifixion. Hyssop, commonly used in herbal medicine, was used to cleanse houses. Additionally, the Rose of Sharon, used to treat itchy skin and other skin problems, was mentioned in the Song of Solomon. There are dozens of other essential oils explicitly stated in the Bible, but they are all referred to as being rejuvenating and having the ability to "rejoice the heart."

When it comes to essential oils, one of the most vital inventions was the process of distillation. Distillation is the process by which certain substances are separated from a liquid. For essential oils, this means getting the actual oil separated from the plant. A technique for distillation was invented during the golden age of the

Arabs, which is predicted to have occurred from the 8th century to the 14th century. The Arabs' experienced a breakthrough when they successfully extracted ethyl alcohol from fermented sugar. Their newfound process of distillation provided them with an easier, faster, and more efficient method of obtaining the valuable oils found within oil-producing vegetation.

During this period of exponential growth for the Arabs, chemist Al-Kindi was an indispensable source of knowledge and innovation. Dubbed the "father of Arab philosophy," Al-Kindi (née Abu Yūsuf Yaʻqūb ibn ʾIshāq aṣ-Ṣabbāḥ al-Kindī) wrote what would become a staple for essential oil distillation and instruction: *The Book of Gentleness on Perfume*, otherwise known as *The Book of the Chemistry of Perfume and Distillations*. This chemist's guide to all things perfumes and essential oils contained perfume recipes, instructions for extracting different oils from plants, and descriptions of distillation tools and techniques. In addition to making important discoveries in the field of medicine, Al-Kindi has also been attributed with advancements in the fields of mathematics, optics, and music theory.

Persian chemist Avicenna, who also went by the names Abu Ali Sina and Ibn Sina, is another polymath whose work played an integral role during the Islamic Golden Age, especially when it came to the chemistry behind essential oils. His works *The Book of Healing* and *The Canon of Medicine* greatly influenced the field of medicine, and he was widely praised within the world of medical academia. In regards to essential oils, Avicenna was the first person to use distillation as a means of extracting the attar of roses, commonly referred to as rose oil, from rose petals. Avicenna then went on to use advanced steam distillation as a way of producing rose essence, which he used to aid in the treatment of various heart conditions.

Ibn al-Baiter (née Ḍiyā' Al-Dīn Abū Muḥammad ʿAbdllāh Ibn Aḥmad al-Mālaqī) was another notable thinker of the Islamic

Golden Age and Arab Agricultural Revolution. Thanks to al-Baiter, the medicine used during the Middle Ages was recorded and kept safe for hundreds of years, making it possible to track the historical use of medicine throughout time. In one of his works, Ibn al-Baiter details the process behind the production of both rosewater and orange water: "The scented Shurub (Syrup) was often extracted from flowers and rare leaves, by means of using hot oils and fat, they were later cooled in cinnamon oil. The oils used were also extracted from sesame and olives. Essential oil was produced by joining various retorts, the steam from these retorts condensed, combined and its scented droplets were used as perfume and mixed to produce the most costly medicines."

The knowledge surrounding essential oils continued to grow and expand during the Middle Ages, a period in European history that lasted until 1520. During this time period of cultural importance, the Catholic Church declared that essential oils were satanic and unnatural. Anyone who used essential oils as a form of medicine or otherwise was accused of being a witch. The English Medieval Witchcraft Acts of 1541, 1562, and 1603 forbade the "use devise practise or exercise, or cause to be devysed practised or exercised, any Invovacons or cojuracons of Sprites witchecraftes enchauntementes or sorceries to thentent to fynde money or treasure or to waste consume or destroy any person in his bodie membres, or to pvoke [provoke] any persone to unlawfull love, or for any other unlawfull intente or purpose." In case you don't speak medieval English, essential oils were viewed as an unlawful method of witchcraft, so for many years those who used essential oils kept it a secret.

As more people became educated in the benefits and purposes of essential oils, there were fewer associations of essential oils with witchcraft and more associations of essential oils with science and medicine. The increased acceptance of essential oils was ushered in by scientists and chemists that were dedicated to teaching the world about their newly discovered remedies. English herbalist John Gerard was one of those people. Gerard lived from 1545-1612 and contributed crucial findings and research to the field of botany. His book titled *Herball* is an encyclopedia of plants and contains descriptions and drawings of over 1000 types of herbs. Though there has been debate over how much of *Herball* is Gerard's original work, the book itself proved extremely helpful when it came to advancing botanical fields during the Middle Ages.

In his thirty-seven years on Earth, Nicholas Culpeper made significant contributions to the fields of botany, herbology, medicine, and astrology. The Cambridge-educated scholar established his own pharmacy, where he often used herbs to treat his patients' illnesses. His use of oils and herbs led to him being accused of witchcraft, which prompted the Worshipful Society of Apothecaries to warn Culpeper against continuing his practice. Radical for his time, Culpeper continued to provide herbal services to his community, often free of charge. He helped to spread the use of herbal remedies by selling his work titled *The English Physician*, which was the first medical book published in the American colonies, for a cheap price. He famously said, "Three kinds of people mainly disease the people – priests, physicians and lawyers – priests disease matters belonging to their souls, physicians disease matters belonging to their bodies, and lawyers disease matters belonging to their estate." Some of the medicinal herbs and plants popularized by Culpeper include fennel, basil, thyme, mint, and sage.

French chemist Rene-Maurice Gattefosse coined the term "aromatherapy" in the 1920s. The word first appeared in his book *Aromathérapie: Les Huiles Essentielles, Hormones Végétales*. Gattefosse discovered the healing properties of lavender oil on accident. He burned his hand and, in an act of desperation, doused the burn in the nearest liquid, which happened to be lavender oil. He later detailed the instance in his own words: "The external application of small quantities of essences rapidly stops the spread of gangrenous sores. In my personal experience, after a laboratory explosion covered me with burning substances which I extinguished by rolling on a grassy lawn, both my hands were covered with a rapidly developing gas gangrene. Just one rinse with lavender essence stopped 'the gasification of the tissue'. This treatment was followed by profuse sweating, and healing began the next day."

Austrian biochemist Madame Marguerite Maury was another pioneer of aromatherapy. A student of Rene-Maurice Gattefosse, Maury took much of Gattefosse's research and expanded it, delving deeper than ever before into the mysteries of essential oils. Though her identity as a woman in a predominately male-dominated field led to a few obstacles, Maury broke through any barriers that impeded her path to scientific discovery. In 1961, she published *Marguerite Maury's Guide To Aromatherapy: The Secret Of Life And Youth*, which wasn't met with critical acclaim until its subsequent release in Britain three years later, in 1964. *The Secret of Life* contains research invaluable to the essential oils market and details ways in which essential oils and other substances can be used to enhance all areas of life. Maury also popularized aromatherapy massage, stressing the idea that good energies and the external application of essential oils can lead to a less stressful, more youthful life. Maury worked on her research and writings up until her last day. Literally. She had been working on her final manuscript, which was found beside her bed when she died on September 25th, 1968. The first sentence read, "The aromatherapy involved in cosmetology can lead to the most extraordinary of results."

Frenchman Dr. Jean Valnet was serving as an army surgical assistant in the Indo-China war when he discovered just how powerful essential oils could be. When his unit ran out of the usual antiseptic medical supplies, one of which was a dangerous compound known as carbolic acid, Dr. Valnet was forced to use essential oils to treat the soldiers' wounds. As it turns out, the essential oils did just a good of a job - if not a better one - at eradicating infections.

Dr. Valnet took the knowledge he had learned during his time in the war and applied it to his clinical practice, where he often used essential oils during surgeries. After conducting an extensive amount of research, Dr. Valnet discovered that essential oils could be used to treat psychiatric disorders such as depression, bipolar affective disorder, and anxiety. He became the first doctor to use essential oils to treat these types of issues. In 1964, Dr. Valnet published his findings in *The Practice of Aromatherapy: A Classic Compendium of Plant Medicines and Their Healing Properties*, a manual that wasn't published in the United States until 1980. In *The Practice of Aromatherapy*, Dr. Valney advocates for the increased use of natural remedies rather than the chemicals commonly found in modern medicine, insisting that, despite the fact that there was still a long way to go in terms of explaining how essential oils work, "There is nothing less scientific than to deny something because it cannot be explained."

An extensive amount of research regarding essential oils has been conducted since the 1980s. Essential oils have been proven to be effective when it comes to treating a variety of illnesses and health complications, and the different uses of essential oils have been taught in medical schools around the world.

Due to a spike in popularity, the essential oils market has become quite saturated in recent years. It can be intimidating if you're new to the world of essential oils, so here are a few essential oil brands that we recommend based on their quality, purity, and price.

YOUNG LIVING

Young Living was founded by Donald Gary Young, the "father of the modern-day essential oils movement," in 1993. D. Gary Young and his wife, Mary Young, started concocting oils on their essential oil distillery and herb farm. They quickly perfected their techniques and expanded their operation, eventually becoming the largest essential oil distillery in North America. The Young Living Headquarters is located in Lehi, Utah, and has offices around the world.

Young Living uses a multi-level marketing business model, which means that there are employees tasked with going out into the world and finding customers individually. This means that, for the most part, you're going to have to find a Young Living ambassador in order to purchase any of the products. These employees are very knowledgeable about the oils and get a commission on all of their sales.

Young Living is the brand that introduced me to the world of essential oils. Young Living is very beginner-friendly. They offer guides for people new to essential oils that include information on how essential oils work, where the oils come from, and different ways to incorporate the oils into your daily routine.

Young Living is proud to offer the highest quality oils, vowing to abide by a special Seed to Seal decree that focuses on sourcing, science, and standards. Young Living's mission is to "enhance and empower lives around the world by sharing the unique benefits of nature's living energy–essential oils," and their commitment to customer service and essential oil quality certainly reflects that.

The prices of Young Living essential oils are not cheap. You're going to pay higher prices for higher quality oils. Young Living's starter kits cost around $160 and are available on Amazon.com or through a Young Living seller. They even offer essential oils for pets, called Animal Scents, that go for around $36 per bottle.

PLANT THERAPY

Plant Therapy is one of the fastest-growing essential oil brands out there. The company was founded by businessman Chris Jones, who attributes his interest in essential oils to his mother, who was an aromatherapist. Plant Therapy offers a wide range of essential oils, including singles, blends, and KidSafe options. Plant Therapy prides itself on its quality ingredients, affordable pricing, and philanthropic efforts. Their oils are both USDA certified and Leaping Bunny certified, which means that their products are organic and cruelty-free.

Two of the big draws of Plant Therapy are its KidSafe oils and its Oil of the Month Club. Plant Therapy's KidSafe essential oils are the first oils developed with the sole purpose of being safe for children. Plant Therapy ensures that their KidSafe oils are both safe and effective: "Our groundbreaking KidSafe blends are specifically formulated for children ages two and up. Our KidSafe line features various blends and single oils targeted toward specific issues and concerns common in this age range. All our blends are available as 100% pure, undiluted essential oils, with several available as convenient pre-diluted roll-ons," says the Plant Therapy website. "As parents ourselves, the Plant Therapy team wouldn't settle for anything less than absolute safety. Our aromatherapists dedicated themselves to research, testing, and quality assurance to make our KidSafe line is unparalleled in the industry."

Plant Therapy's Oil of the Month Club delivers a unique mystery oil blend to your door every month. You can become a member for $15 a month or sign up as a one-time buyer for $20. The sizes of the oils range from 2.5 mL to 30 mL. Previous oils of the month include wild chrysanthemum absolute, balm mint bush, and hinoki leaf.

Plant Therapy is much more affordable than Young Living. Their most popular kit contains seven single oils and seven synergies for $60, and their KidSafe starter kit will cost you $50.

REVIVE ESSENTIAL OILS

Revive Essential Oils was founded by CEO Alexandria George and is run by her and her family. A newer essential oil company, Revive's guarantee states, "We use REVIVE Essential Oils every day ourselves, with our kids and families. We love REVIVE Essential Oils and think you will too. We're so confident, we offer free returns. Simply return your opened or unopened bottles for a full refund within 100 days of purchase, no questions asked. We pay the cost of return shipping too."

Revive's essential oils are 100% pure, bottled in the United States, and are free of harmful fillers such as synthetic linalool and synthetic linalyl acetate. Their oils are also cruelty-free and sustainably sourced, making them safe for people, animals, and the planet. Revive Essential Oils also makes sure to provide beginners with the knowledge they need in order to understand how to use their oils. When I first opened the Revive website, a window popped up and asked if I would like to be emailed a "Top 50 Uses of Essential Oils" guide to further familiarize myself with the many benefits of essential oils.

One of the biggest perks of choosing Revive Essential Oils over a company like Young Living is that Revive doesn't follow the multi-level marketing business model, which means that Revive's essential oils will be much more affordable than those of Young Living. "REVIVE is sold directly from our website and delivered to your door. We don't have any middlemen selling our product. Those middlemen are expensive and make essential oils more expensive for you. We sell directly to you which means we can have the same high-quality essential oils but sell them at a cheaper price because we are passing on the savings directly to you," says Revive's website.

The Revive essential oil starter kit costs $85 and includes ten full-sized bottles of their best-selling blends: Lavender, Lemon, Peppermint, Tea Tree, Frankincense, Copaiba, Immunity Boost, Sleep, Breathe Air, and Stress Easy. If you buy from Revive and aren't happy with your purchase, it's no problem. Revive Essential Oils offers a 100% money-back guarantee for both opened and unopened bottles.

EDENS GARDEN

Edens Garden is a women-owned and operated business that was founded by Grace Martin in 2009. Martin began working in the natural industry in 2002, but it wasn't until she was on an eye-opening mission trip in New Zealand that she decided to start what would become Edens Garden. "I would explore the island, picking flowers and plants and pressing them in books to share with friends," says Martin. "Incredibly pure, clean, and fresh, I learned that essential oils offer that same refreshing and captivating experience of nature, and I again wanted to share that sense of calm."

Since its inception, Edens Garden has sold over 20 million bottles and received more than one million five-star reviews. Eden Garden's oils are sustainably made, cruelty-free, vegan, and are GC/MS batch-tested to ensure safe use. Like Revive Essential Oils, Edens Garden sells its products directly to the consumer, cutting out the middleman as well as the price. Edens Garden's pledge is as follows: "We are dedicated to making natural and effective essential oil products for you, our customer, while providing education about how to safely enjoy their benefits."

Edens Garden offers essential oil roll-ons, diamond and stone diffusers, and diffuser bracelets, which you can add drops of oil to in order to transport your favorite essential oils with you wherever you go. The bracelets cost $40, and the diffusers range from

$65 to $75. Another attractive feature provided by Edens Garden is the Blend of the Month. Each month, Edens Garden sells a limited-edition oil blend. July's Blend of the Month is Malibu Cove, a perfect summer oil with a tropical and citrusy aroma.

The 3-piece Best of the Best Essential Oil set costs $22 and includes the Fighting Five Blend, Lavender, and Lemon oils. Edens Garden also provides an option to create your own essential oil set. If you choose to purchase this set, you'll be given the chance to curate a set of 3, 6, 12, 24, or 48 essential oils. The custom sets range from $21 to $300.

DOTERRA

doTERRA was founded in 2008 by a group of healthcare and business professionals. doTERRA is a Latin word that means "Gift of the Earth." In order to ensure that their oils are 100% pure, doTERRA established the CPTG Certified Pure Tested Grade® protocol, which involves "a rigorous examination of every batch of oil, along with third-party testing to guarantee transparency."

Like Young Living, doTERRA utilizes the multi-level marketing business model, where consumers work with Wellness Advocates in order to discover which essential oils would best fit their needs. In addition to essential oil blends, doTERRA's website sells hair care supplies, weight management supplements, and portable oil diffusers.

doTERRA's commitment to sustainability is evident in two of the essential oil company's initiatives: Co-Impact Sourcing and the doTERRA Healing Hands Foundation. Co-Impact Sourcing ensures that the production process of doTERRA's oils is ethically sound and completely transparent. "Our Co-Impact Sourcing model for essential oils effectively integrates our business model with our philanthropic priorities as a company," says Vice President of doTERRA's Global Strategic Sourcing Tim Valentiner. "We believe that a key part of international development is, and will continue to be, carried out by businesses that see the return on investment for social impact programs linked to the sourcing or manufacturing of their products from developing countries."

The doTERRA Healing Hands Foundation is a nonprofit "seeking to empower communities worldwide to make a sustainable change by supporting initiatives that alleviate extreme poverty, improve quality of life, and ensure basic human rights." Some of their initiatives include HOPE (Anti-Human Trafficking), disaster relief, and women empowerment. The Healing Hands Foundation has impacted nearly 70 countries around the world, distributed over 120,000 emergency relief hygiene kits, and completed 180 projects. The nonprofit celebrated its 10-year anniversary in June 2020.

doTERRA's Introductory Kit contains three 5 mL bottles of their most popular essential oils: Lavender, Lemon, and Peppermint. It also comes with a guide that lists some helpful essential oil tips and tricks. The Introductory Kit costs $26.67 and is a perfect starting point for essential oil newbies.

doTERRA's Global Corporate Headquarters is located in Pleasant Grove, Utah and is run by current CEO David Stirling.

Each company that we've listed comes with a unique set of pros and cons. Whether you choose to purchase your essential oils from Young Living, Revive, Plant Therapy, Edens Garden, doTERRA, or some other essential oil company, you'll be in good hands when it comes to beginning your essential oil journey.

BUT BEFORE YOU BEGIN…

While these essential oils are beneficial, they are also quite strong. It is crucial that when you use them for topical purposes, always use a carrier oil like coconut or jojoba oil. These carrier oils help to dilute essential oils. You should also do a patch test before applying this to any part of your body in case you are allergic or sensitive to the product.

Very few essential oils can be taken orally; however, not all are like this. When ingesting orally, you should either place the drops of oil into a gel capsule and drink it with water or add the drops directly to about a cup of liquid, possibly milk or water, before drinking. Before taking in any essential oils, please check with your healthcare professional and find out which ones are safe to ingest.

Always, and we can't stress this enough, always buy essential oils that are labeled as "pure." There are many knock-off versions in the market that do not carry any benefits. So be mindful of what product you are purchasing.

TYPES OF ESSENTIAL OILS

As you have probably seen, there is not just one essential oil out there. Each of these scents has their own benefits. Whether you're suffering from skin problems, nausea, or low self-esteem, there's an essential oil out there that will fit your needs. Each essential oil that is included in our guide has been tested through various studies, some of which we've briefly described and referenced below. Here are a few of the most common essential oils in the market currently:

Lavender Oil

This essential oil has a subtle floral scent and is best known for its calming benefits. Lavender has been around for ages and is used to treat many types of ailments such as anxiety, insomnia, depression, hair loss, nausea, acne, skin irritations, etc. It is most commonly used in aromatherapy as its fragrance promotes calmness. In addition to all of the benefits of lavender when it comes to the skin, lavender oil also has benefits in other areas of life. For example, lavender oil works as an effective insect repellent. Just add a few drops of lavender oil to any candle to turn it into instant bug repellant. There are many ways to use this product such as by inhaling it through an aromatherapy diffuser, applying it to your skin, adding it to your bath, spraying it on your pillows, etc.

I first used lavender oil after burning my hand on the stove. After I told my mom that I had burned my hand, she practically jumped up and down. "I just bought something that might help," she said. My mom then made a beeline for the pantry. When she came back, she was holding a small glass bottle labeled "Plant Therapy: Lavender Oil." She took my burned hand and put on a drop of the oil. I instantly felt cool relief spread over my burned skin. I was surprised. What was this liquid and why did it smell so good? "Apply this lavender oil every day, and then let me know if it's working," said my mom. And it did work. A few days later, the burn had completely healed, as if it were never even there in the first place.

WARNING – Despite its many benefits, lavender oil does have a few side effects: nausea, headaches, skin irritations (for those with sensitive skin), and vomiting. Always check with your general physician before getting in contact with the oil.

Rose Oil

Rose essential oil is great for reducing anxiety, treating acne, and even imposing skin complexion to a certain extent. It is extracted from the petals of various Rosa species such as *Rosa centifolia* L. and *Rosa damascena* Mill. It's important to check the rose oil bottles to see which plant the rose oil is extracted from. Many studies have found that rose oil does in fact have many therapeutic properties such as functioning as analgesics and anti-depressants. Based on Persian Medicine, it has a few other pharmacological features such as being anti-inflammatory and anti-hemorrhoidal.

In a 2013 study, rose oil was tested for its effects on menstrual pain. There were two groups: a group that was given almond oil and a group that was given a mixture of almond oil and rose oil. In this case, almond oil was the carrier oil, which means that its purpose is to help dilute the essential oil so that it is most effective on your skin. Both menstruating groups were then massaged with their respective oils. The group that was massaged with rose oil reported lower levels of menstrual discomfort than did the purely almond oil group, supporting the idea that rose oil can be used to help ease period cramps.

An experiment conducted by the Iran University of Medical Sciences tested rose oil's effectiveness in reducing anxiety for women in labor. There were three groups in this study. The first group was given a 10-minute inhalation and warm foot bath infused with rose oil. The second group was given a plain footbath with warm water. The third group served as the control group and went through birthing procedures as they usually would. The women's anxiety was then measured using the visual analogous scale (VAS). The results of the study showed that women were significantly less anxious after the rose oil footbath than with any of the other footbaths. The study made sure to point out the link between rose oil and the women's lessened anxiety: "Rose scent is effective on the central nervous system. Two materials, sytrinol and 2-phenyl ethyl alcohol, in roses are known as antianxiety agents. Using oil rose reduces anxiety by 71% in labor and only 14% of them need local anesthesia."

Rose oil has also been found to help increase sex drive in patients suffering from a major depressive disorder. Due to the treatments that they undergo for depression, many people who suffer from the major depressive disorder also experience SSRI-induced sexual dysfunctions. In a study affiliated with the Substance Abuse Prevention Research Center, males suffering from depression and low sex drive were instructed to take either Rosa damascena oil or a placebo. They ingested their assigned substances for a month before reporting back to the conductors of the study. The results show more drastically improved SSRI-induced sexual dysfunctions in the men who took rose oil than in the men who took the placebo. Additionally, the men's depression alleviated as their sexual dysfunctions decreased. All of this to show that rose oil works wonders when it comes to decreasing depression and sexual dysfunctions in men, but what about women?

A parallel study was conducted on a group of women suffering from both depression and sexual dysfunctions. The goal of this study was to see if rose oil affected women the same way it affected men who suffered from the same afflictions. Once again, the participants in the study were instructed to take either Rosa damascena or a placebo. Not only did the rose oil decrease the pain associated with sexual dysfunctions, but raking rose oil also increased sexual pleasure.

The best way to use this oil is by inhaling it through a diffuser or by applying it to your chest, neck, and wrists (make sure to dilute it first with a carrier oil). You can also draw a pleasant rose oil bath (or foot bath) by placing about 10 drops of diluted rose oil into a warm tub.

WARNING – The side effects of rose oil include skin irritation. Can be avoided if you increase the amount of the carrier oil; however, if your skin reacts extremely stop using it and see a doctor. Like with most essential oils, it is beneficial to perform a skin patch test before engaging in regular use.

Ylang Ylang Oil

This essential oil has a fruity, yet spicy aroma and is derived from a plant that grows on the Cananga tree. It has been a staple in the market for years. It has a long list of benefits for your health such as promoting relaxation, reducing depression, killing bacteria, lowering blood pressure, sexual stimulation, improving memory, and building self-esteem. It is often found in many cosmetic products because of its beauty benefits.

A Universidade de São Paulo study found evidence that supported the idea that ylang ylang is effective for boosting self-esteem. The participants in the study were split up into three groups. The first group received ylang ylang oil topically. The second group inhaled ylang ylang oil. The final group received a placebo. Throughout the duration of the study, the participants were asked to rate their self-esteem on the Dela Coleta self-esteem scale. Participants who took ylang ylang oil either by means of inhalation or directly on their skin showed signs of increased self-esteem, whereas the participants who were given the placebo did not. Of course, there are many external factors that could have caused the participants' increased self-esteem, but most of the signs point to ylang ylang oil as being the biggest contributor.

Ylang Ylang oil has also been used to successfully treat head lice in children, though more research needs to be conducted before ylang ylang is officially accepted as a cure for head lice.

Ylang ylang oil can be added to baths, applied to the skin, and even inhaled through an oil diffuser.

WARNING – Side effects include skin irritation, poisonous to dogs and cats, has few ingredients that people may be allergic to. Ylang ylang contains isoeugenol, which is an allergen, so it is suggested to consult with a health professional before use.

Peppermint Oil

Peppermint oil is one of the most popular essential oils on the market. The minty oil has been used since ancient times. Peppermint essential oil has a minty herbal aroma and is best used for boosting your energy levels, improving digestion, relieving pain, reducing vomiting sensations and irritable bowel syndrome, soothing muscle spasms, etc.

A meta-analysis (a conglomeration of multiple scientific studies) authored by The Johns Hopkins University School of Medicine explored the effect of peppermint oil on irritable bowel syndrome, a chronic gastrointestinal (GI) condition that causes diarrhea, constipation, and other internal issues. The meta-analysis took data found in studies done by MEDLINE (PubMed), Cochrane Central Register of Controlled Trials (Cochrane CENTRAL), ClinicalTrials.gov, EMBASE (Ovid), and Web of Science in order to summarize the ways in which peppermint oil has affected people suffering from irritable bowel syndrome. The meta-analysis included 12 trials and 835 patients. "PO contains L-menthol, which blocks calcium channels in smooth muscle, thus producing antispasmodic effects on the gastrointestinal tract," wrote the meta-analysis authors. "PO possesses antimicrobial, anti-inflammatory, antioxidant, immunomodulating, and anesthetic activities, all of which may be relevant for the treatment of IBS." The conclusions of the meta-analysis supported the notion that peppermint oil is very effective and undoubtedly safe when it comes to treating irritable bowel syndrome.

Peppermint oil is also effective when it comes to treating functional dyspepsia, another chronic gastrointestinal condition. According to the Mayo Clinic, functional dyspepsia symptoms include "upper abdominal discomfort, described as burning sensation, bloating or gassiness, nausea, or feeling full too quickly after starting to eat." A scientific review suggests that peppermint oil, when used in conjunction with caraway oil, is a competent reliever of IBS and functional dyspepsia symptoms. The problem with this method, however, is that caraway oil hasn't been proven safe for individuals under the age of 18.

A different review was written on children and adolescents who have experienced gastronomical complications. The review conductors collected data from fourteen trials and 1,927 trial participants before reaching their conclusion: "when compared with the placebo, peppermint oil significantly reduced the duration of pain (minutes/day), frequency of pain (episodes per week), and severity of pain. In comparison with probiotics, peppermint oil significantly reduced the duration of pain (minutes/day) and the severity of pain."

Another one of peppermint oil's many uses is for the treatment of nausea. Patricia Briggs, Helen Hawrylack, and Ruth Mooney were the authors of a study that investigated the effects of peppermint oil on postoperative patients. Postoperative patients commonly experience uncomfortable nausea, and the drugs usually administered to treat nausea have adverse side effects. The authors of the study wanted to see if peppermint oil could serve as a safer, yet still effective, alternative to these antiemetics. The results were as follows: "The average nausea rating before the use of peppermint oil was 3.29 (SD, 1.0) on a scale of 0 to 5, with 5 being the greatest nausea. Two minutes later, the average nausea rating was 1.44 (SD, 1.3). Using paired t-tests, these differences were found to be statistically significant (P = 0.000)." In conclusion, peppermint oil significantly helped to reduce nausea following medical operations, making it a viable option for patients who want to get rid of nausea without the possibility of the usual negative side effects.

Because nausea and stomach-related issues are also associated with pregnancy, peppermint oil has been suggested as a treatment for pregnant women. Studies have shown, however, that there is virtually no difference between peppermint oil and the placebo when it comes to easing nausea in pregnant women.

In general, peppermint oil has been shown to help with pain management. There are three studies that back the claim that peppermint oil can help relieve pain in different areas of the body. The first study, affiliated with the Comparative Medicine Research Center and Department of Neurology, investigated the effect of peppermint oil on headaches and migraines. The study participants were divided into two groups: a menthol group and a placebo group. Menthol is the active ingredient in peppermint. The menthol and placebo substances were applied topically across the participants' foreheads. The participants were then asked to fill out questionnaires related to the amount of pain they were feeling. After the study concluded and the questionnaires were turned in, the results ruled in favor of peppermint oil. It was concluded that "menthol solution can be an efficacious, safe and tolerable therapeutic option for the abortive treatment of migraine."

Monitored by the Jefferson Headache Center, the second study sought to discover the effects that peppermint oil and its active ingredient menthol have on migraine attacks. The participants in the study had to have been diagnosed by the International Classification of Headache Disorders with episodic migraines for at least one year prior. In order to be eligible for the study, patients had to have suffered at least one severe migraine per month. Over the course of 8 weeks, participants applied the menthol gel and wrote about their migraine experiences in a diary. The results were as follows: "Prior to treatment, 7 patients had mild pain, 13 moderate pain, and 5 severe pain. Two hours following gel application, 7 (28%) patients had no pain, 7 (28%) mild pain, 6 (25%) moderate pain, and 5 (20%) severe pain. The majority of patients had similar pain intensity (8; 32%) or improvement (13; 52%). At 24-h, only two non-rescued patients still had a mild headache." These observations support the idea that peppermint oil is effective at relieving pain associated with migraines.

The final study was conducted in 2019 and explored the effects of peppermint oil on dysphagia and chest pain that is caused by esophageal motility disorders. Researchers at the Medical University of South Carolina's Division of Gastroenterology and Hepatology believed that peppermint oil's smooth muscle relaxing properties could have a positive impact on people who experience chest pain and other related conditions. Study participants were instructed to ingest peppermint tablets in intervals throughout the day. Afterwards, they responded to questions using the five-point Likert scale, which records the participants' levels of agreement (strongly disagree, disagree, neither agree nor disagree, etc.) regarding a set of statements. "Peppermint Oil appears to provide symptomatic relief in some patients with dysphagia and Chest Pain," concludes the study's authors. "Presence of a well-defined manometric disorder, particularly DES or EGJOO, appeared to predict response."

The benefits of peppermint oil extend beyond internal issues. Peppermint oil has also been confirmed to help with skin problems such as itchiness and irritation. A study carried out by the Department of Dermatology at Al Azhar University in Egypt tested a 1% peppermint oil solution on people who have been diagnosed with chronic pruritus, which, according to the Mayo Clinic, is an "an uncomfortable, irritating sensation that creates an urge to scratch that can involve any part of the body." The itchiness before and after peppermint oil application was measured via the 5-D itch scale (5D-IS). After the study had reached its end, the researchers had reached a conclusion: "The topical treatment of chronic pruritus with peppermint oil is effective, easy to use, safe, cheap, and more acceptable for those whose topical and systemic treatments tend to be irritating, contraindicated, or less well tolerated."

As you can tell by the plethora of studies listed above, peppermint oil is extremely versatile and effective when it comes to improving a variety of health concerns. Peppermint oil can be applied to the skin, used in an oil diffuser, put in the bath, and sprayed on sheets. Ingesting pure peppermint oil is dangerous and not recommended.

WARNING – Side effects include heartburn, headaches, mouth sores, vomiting, and irritated esophagus if ingested. Peppermint oil can be dangerous if taken in large doses. It contains a harmful toxin called pulegone, which is a naturally occurring insecticide that is poisonous to rats (and humans). Pregnant women and children should use caution when using peppermint oil, as it could have adverse health effects. As always, it's vital to dilute your essential oils with a carrier oil before use in order to ensure safety.

Tea Tree Oil

Also known as melaleuca oil, tea tree oil is derived from the Australian tea tree. Although tea tree oil has been recognized for its antibacterial and soothing properties since ancient times, the name "Tea Tree" wasn't coined until 1770, when British explorer Captain James Cook observed native Australians using the leaves of the Melaleuca alternifolia to make an aromatic tea. The Aboriginal Australians would use the tea tree leaves to cure colds and coughs, heal cuts and wounds, and aid in the treatment of many other problems. During World War II, soldiers would even carry tea tree oil in their medical kits to treat wounded soldiers.

This is another common and highly used essential oil that has numerous benefits. Tea tree oil is best for soothing allergic skin reactions or inflammations, treating dandruff, reducing hair loss, stimulating blood circulation, serving as a natural hand sanitizer, and even improving acne-prone skin. There are recipes online for homemade tea tree insect spray, soap, disinfectant spray, air purifier, and toothbrush cleaner.

Tea tree oil can treat a number of common skin concerns such as oily skin, acne, psoriasis, cuts and skin wounds, inflammation, and hair and scalp treatment. Participants in a 2016 study wore tea tree oil-infused sunscreen to see how it affected their oily skin. The results of the study showed significant improvements in "oiliness, porphyrins, hydration and desquamation."

In a study conducted by the Skin Diseases and Leishmaniasis Research Center, it was confirmed that tea tree oil is an effective solution for acne vulgaris, which is simply the more specific term for general acne. The clinical trial was performed on 60 people who have experienced mild to moderate acne. The participants were divided into two groups. One group was instructed to apply 5% tea tree gel onto their problem areas. The other group was given a placebo. The study lasted 45 days, and the study conductors checked in with the participants every 15 days. During the check-ins, the participants tracked their skin condition by using the total acne lesions counting (TLC) and acne severity index (ASI). By the end of the study, the people who had used tea tree oil to treat their acne showed significant improvement in their skin condition, while those that had used the placebo didn't experience much of a difference.

But how does tea tree oil compare to something like benzoyl peroxide, one of the most popular acne treatments on the market? The Department of Dermatology at the Royal Prince Alfred Hospital conducted a study to find out. The study was comprised of 124 participants and compared the effects of 5% tea tree oil gel and 5% benzoyl peroxide. The results of the study showed similar acne improvements for the tea tree oil gel users and the benzoyl peroxide users. However, those that used benzoyl peroxide to treat their acne experienced faster results than those that used tea tree oil gel. On the other hand, the tea tree oil gel users experienced fewer negative side effects. There are pros and cons to each treatment option, so it all depends on personal preference.

You can use peppermint oil in an oil diffuser or apply it topically. It has been proven to be safe for external use, but ingesting tea tree oil should be avoided, as it could cause blackouts, lack of muscle control, and confusion.

Lemon Oil

Lemon oil was utilized by ancient civilizations in places like Asia, Egypt, and Rome to treat diseases. Lemon trees are native to Asia. They were introduced to Europeans in 200 A.D. and were ultimately brought to America by Christopher Columbus. Lemon oil was also used in Ayurvedic medicine, one of the world's most ancient medical and healing systems.

A citrusy essential oil filled with many antioxidant properties that reduce inflammation, help treat anemia, boost energy, relieve headaches, and improve digestion. Lemon oil can be used as a non-toxic alternative to chemical-heavy household cleaners. It can also help with delaying the tarnishing of silver as well as the preservation of leather furniture.

According to a 2006 stress test study that was published in PubMed Central, lemon essential oil helped a group of mice calm down and stabilize their moods. Similar calming effects of lemon oil have been found in humans, and studies have been published that show evidence of lemon oil reducing depression and anxiety in adults.

Lemon oil has been proven to be an effective combatant against bacteria Staphylococcus aureus and Escherichia coli, which means that it can be used to clean small wounds. Finally, lemon oil could possibly aid in relieving nausea. In a study conducted on pregnant women, lemon oil was reported to have decreased morning sickness and vomiting. Lemon oil's bright aroma can provide an uplifting boost and replenish one's energy throughout the day.

In vitro and in vivo research - research carried out in a laboratory and usually involving the study of microorganisms - completed in 2018 aimed to assess the efficacy of lemon oil on skin inflammation. After the study was finished, the researchers at the CSIR-Central Institute of Medicinal and Aromatic Plants concluded that lemon oil does indeed show promising signs of serving as an effective treatment for skin inflammation.

Lemon oil can also be used to aid in concentration and alertness. The Faculty of Education at Firat Üniversitesi in Elazig, Turkey tested lemon oil on a group of 58 primary school children to see how it affected their English language test performance. It turns out that lemon oil had a positive effect on the children's test scores. The study group that received lemon oil treatment earned higher mean scores than the study group that didn't receive lemon oil treatment. The results of the study supported the idea that lemon oil improves students' concentration, alertness, and retention rate: "The use of lemon essence oil aroma as an olfactory stimulus was found to be associated with improved achievement. Furthermore, the retention rate of pupils who had been exposed to the stimulus exceeded that of a control group."

You can either use lemon oil in an oil diffuser or apply it topically. It's important to operate the diffuser in a ventilated area and to always apply the lemon essential oil with a carrier oil.

WARNING – Because this oil is highly photosensitive, avoid any exposure to sunlight after applying it to your skin. It is better to use it at night and wash it in the morning. One of the potential side effects is the experience of a burning sensation on the skin. It is highly recommended that you test the lemon oil on a patch of skin to see if any reactions occur before routine use.

Eucalyptus Oil

First used by Australian Aborigines, eucalyptus oil is extracted from the leaves of the eucalyptus tree and used to treat many common ailments such as coughs, stuffy noses, fevers, muscle pain, and joint pain. Eucalyptus oil has a sweet minty aroma that some have compared to Vicks VapoRub, which makes it perfect for giving your sinuses a wake-up call.

Like all of the previously listed essential oils, eucalyptus oil has been tested in various scientific studies for its efficacy. In a study monitored by the Department of Basic Nursing Science of Korea University, eucalyptus oil was tested for its effects on pain and inflammation in total knee replacement patients. In the clinical trial, the participants were randomly placed in either a eucalyptus oil inhalation group or an almond oil inhalation group. The participants rated their pain on a visual analog scale (VAS) before and after inhalation of the essential oil. Over the course of the study, the VAS scores for those who had inhaled eucalyptus oil decreased, while the VAS scores for those who had inhaled almond oil increased. The results of the study were in favor of eucalyptus oil: "In summary, this study, which investigated the effects of eucalyptus oil inhalation on patients who underwent TKR, showed that eucalyptus oil inhalation was effective in reducing patient's subjective pain and blood pressure after surgery. These findings suggest that the inhalation of eucalyptus oil might be a valuable nursing intervention for pain relief after TKR."

Eucalyptus oil can be taken internally by adults. Dilute the oil in warm water before ingesting it. Eucalyptus oil can also be boiled and steeped with water to make tea. If you're using the eucalyptus oil to heal a wound, add a few drops to any petroleum jelly and apply generously on the affected areas. You can also add drops to a diffuser for inhalation.

WARNING - Eucalyptus oil may cause an allergic reaction, so be sure to conduct a patch test before use. Always dilute eucalyptus oil before use. Not diluting your eucalyptus essential oil can cause dizziness, stomach pain, vomiting, fatigue, and, in cases where undiluted oil dosage exceeds a teaspoon, death.

Frankincense Oil

Frankincense oil is derived from five different species of frankincense tree, two of the most common being *Boswellia carterii* and *B. freraeana*. Dubbed the "king of oils," frankincense oil has been around since ancient times. Frankincense was traded on the Silk Road, researched by ancient Greek historian Gerodotus, and given to baby Jesus as a birthday present. It can be used to reduce arthritis, soothe inflamed skin, improve oral health, and improve both focus and relaxation. Frankincense oil has a musky, earthy scent comparable to rosemary.

There have been many studies testing the effectiveness and adequacy of eucalyptus oil. However, when it comes to certain claims, such as the claim that eucalyptus oil can help prevent diabetes, more research needs to be done until they can be considered credible.

One benefit of frankincense oil that is supported by sufficient research is its anti-cancer properties. In a 2017 study affiliated with the Hamadan University of Medical Sciences, Boswellia serrata (Indian frankincense) was tested for its effects on HT-29 colon cancer cells. The results of the study provided evidence that frankincense can be used to slow down the migration, growth, and procreation of colon cancer cells.

Frankincense oil has also been shown to suppress other types of cancers, such as melanoma cancer, prostate cancer, and breast cancer. In addition, research supports the use of frankincense oil in order to reduce the side effects associated with cancer treatment. However, there is still a lot of research that needs to be done before frankincense becomes more widely accepted and confirmed as a cancer remedy.

Frankincense oil can be applied topically or inhaled through a diffuser. Always take extreme caution before ingesting any essential oil.

WARNING - Frankincense oil may cause skin irritation if applied topically. Avoid frankincense oil if you are pregnant or breastfeeding, as it may result in adverse side effects.

Chamomile Oil

Chamomile oil, also referred to as Chamomile Roman, has a sweet and fruity aroma. Ancient Egyptians revered chamomile oil so much that they gifted it to Ra, the god of the sun and the most important god in ancient Egyptian religion. Chamomile oil can help fight depression and anxiety, reduce digestive issues, heal wounds, promote healthy sleep patterns, and decrease muscle pains. Research surrounding chamomile use has increased in recent years, and the results are promising.

If you're like me, you often struggle with getting a good night's sleep. A 2017 study supports the idea that chamomile oil may be able to help with problems related to insomnia. Scientists at the Kashan University of Medical Sciences examined how chamomile oil affects the sleeping patterns of elderly people. The study participants were divided into two groups: a control group and a treatment group. The treatment group was instructed to ingest chamomile capsules twice a day for 28 consecutive days. The control group ingested capsules filled with flour for the same amount of time. By the end of the study, the treatment group reported significantly higher scores on the Sleep Quality Index, which backs the argument that chamomile oil can be used to curb insomnia. Though this study focused solely on people over the age of sixty, it is sufficient to say that chamomile oil would have similar effects for those of younger age groups.

Additional research has proven chamomile oil's benefits when it comes to pain relief, skin irritation, anxiety, and depression. Chamomile oil can be inhaled by means of a diffuser or applied topically. If using topically, be sure to dilute the oil in a carrier oil before applying it to the skin. If you want to ingest chamomile orally, opt for chamomile tea, as consuming chamomile essential oil can have negative side effects.

WARNING - Avoid chamomile oil if you are taking prescription medications, pregnant, or breastfeeding. Chamomile oil may cause skin irritation or allergic reactions, so, as always, conduct a patch test before committing to regular use.

Rosemary Oil

Native to the Mediterranean, rosemary oil has a citrusy, herbal aroma characteristic of its source: *Rosmarinus Officinalis*, a plant that exists in the Mint family. Ancient civilizations used rosemary oil for religious, medical, and cultural purposes. For example, people in the Middle Ages believed that rosemary had the power to stop the spread of the bubonic plague, so they would often keep rosemary in their homes to keep their family members plague-free. Today's uses of rosemary are much more medical and scientifically grounded.

Rosemary oil is said to stimulate hair growth, inhibit skin inflammation, reduce stress and anxiety, repel insects, improve memorization, and relieve pain, among other benefits. Rosemary leaves are most commonly used in cooking and baking, but rosemary oil can replace them in virtually every rosemary-imbued recipe. Just add a few drops of rosemary oil in lieu of the rosemary sprigs and you're good to go!

There have been many studies that have sought to test the efficacy of rosemary oil on many common ailments. For example, researchers at Florida Atlantic University analyzed how rosemary oil affected anxiety-ridden nursing students. The nursing students inhaled either rosemary oil, lavender oil, or no essential oil before taking a test. The participants who inhaled rosemary oil reported increased concentration and reduced anxiety, more so than those who inhaled lavender oil or nothing at all.

Another study tested rosemary oil's effects on androgenetic alopecia, which is a common form of baldness and hair loss. The 2015 study pitted rosemary oil against minoxidil 2%, a common over-the-counter solution for hair loss. Participants were instructed to use either rosemary oil or minoxidil 2%. The findings of the study supported the assertion that rosemary oil is an effective treatment for androgenetic alopecia. Moreover, the participants that used rosemary oil reported less scalp itching than those that used minoxidil 2%.

Rosemary oil can be applied topically in a carrier oil or inhaled through diffusion. Only consume rosemary oil in very small doses, as ingesting too much can have devastating effects.

WARNING - Side effects of rosemary may include internal damage, vomiting, seizures, skin and kidney irritation, and sun sensitivity. Most of these side effects are only possible if you consume the essential oil orally, so take caution if you plan to ingest rosemary oil, especially if you are pregnant or have allergies.

CHOOSING THE RIGHT ESSENTIAL OILS

As we mentioned in the beginning, it is important to check the labels and ingredients of any essential oils before purchasing them. There are numerous companies there who claim to be selling oils that are "pure" or "natural" or "medical grade." But in reality, these terms don't have much credibility in the market. This industry is not regulated, so the quality and the composition of these oils vary.

Here are a few tips to keep in mind the next time you are buying essential oils:

- Quality: Avoid any essential oils that are ridden with excess chemicals. Choose the ones that have been through minimal processing. The best ones are usually extracted through distillation or mechanical cold presses.
- Purity: Always check the ingredient list of the essential oil. make sure that it has only aromatic plant compounds and no additives or synthetics. You know an oil is pure when the ingredient list includes the plant's botanical name and its origin.

> *"If a company does not list the plant's scientific or botanical name as well as where they sourced it from, it's likely not a good product."*

Harpreet Gujral, director of integrative medicine at Sibley Memorial Hospital

- Reputation: Purchase essential oils from reputable companies that are backed by good reviews for creating high-quality essential oils. Any of the companies that we have included in this guide are great options!

AFTERWORD

Hopefully you are now better equipped to purchase essential oils and reap their benefits. The research around the uses of essential oils, especially medically, are still ongoing. But that does not mean that you can't enjoy their amazing and known advantages now. So, this is your sign to take that plunge and join the aromatherapy trend. We promise you won't regret it.

www.ingramcontent.com/pod-product-compliance
Lightning Source LLC
Chambersburg PA
CBHW072236230526
45466CB00024B/2080